THE

TRANSPLANT DIET

RECIPES COOKBOOK

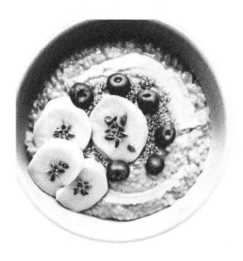

Complete Guide with 50 Low Sodium, Potassium, and Phosphorus Meals to Prevent Complications and Promote Renal Health and Recovery for Transplant Patients

Dixie McCoy

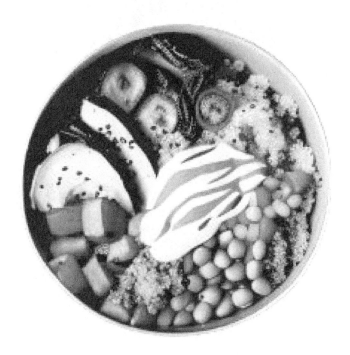

Table of Content

Introduction: Nourishing Your Kidney Health After Transplant Surgery

Imagine, for a moment, the remarkable resiliency of the human body. It is an intricate masterpiece, capable of adaptation and regeneration. Now, consider the profound impact of a kidney transplant—the hope it brings, the second chance at a vibrant life.

Yet, alongside this transformative gift comes a responsibility: the responsibility to nourish and protect this precious organ, to provide it with the sustenance it needs to thrive.

In the wake of a kidney transplant, the relationship between diet and kidney health becomes a cornerstone of recovery. It is no secret that dietary choices exert a profound influence on the body's overall well-being, and this truth becomes especially poignant for transplant recipients.

The right foods can bolster the body's healing process, promote optimal organ function, and enhance vitality.

Within the pages of "The Kidney Transplant Diet Recipes Cookbook", you will discover more than a collection of recipes. This is a culinary companion crafted with a singular mission—to empower individuals recovering from kidney transplant surgery with a treasure trove of delectable and nourishing recipes.

Every recipe within this cookbook is designed not just to tantalize the taste buds, but to elevate kidney health to its zenith. Each ingredient has been meticulously chosen to contribute not only to the flavor profile but to the overarching goal of post-transplant recovery.

In the realm of wellness, food is not merely sustenance; it is medicine. And every meal, a chance to infuse the body with vitality and strength.

As you journey through the pages of "The Kidney Transplant Diet Recipes Cookbook," envision more than just a collection of recipes. Envision a roadmap to a healthier life, a bridge between the culinary and the curative.

Whether you are embarking on this voyage yourself or preparing meals for a loved one who has embraced the gift of a new beginning, rest assured that these recipes have been carefully curated to embrace the needs of post-transplant life.

So, dear reader, as a nutritionist and health cookbook writer, it is my privilege to embark on this journey with you. Let us navigate the world of post-transplant nutrition together, embracing the healing power of food, one delicious recipe at a time.

Therefore, let me welcome you to "The Kidney Transplant Diet Recipes Cookbook." Your nourishing path to renewed vitality after a kidney transplant begins here.

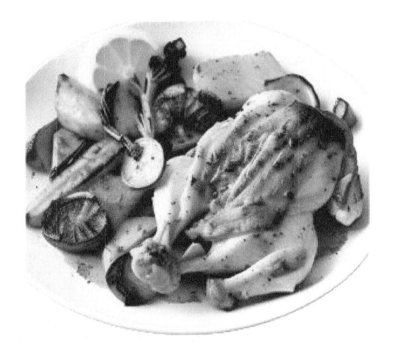

Chapter 1: Understanding Kidney Health and Transplant Recovery

In the journey towards better kidney health and recovery after a kidney transplant, knowledge becomes a potent tool.

This chapter delves into the core principles of kidney health, the crucial significance of post-transplant care, and the pivotal role that diet plays in upholding kidney function and averting potential complications.

Tailored specifically for kidney transplant patients, the insights shared here aim to empower you with essential information to navigate this phase of your life confidently.

The Fundamentals of Kidney Health

Kidneys, those unassuming bean-shaped organs nestled within us, have an astonishingly vital role to play. Their primary function is to filter waste products and excess fluids from the blood, ensuring our bodies maintain a delicate balance.

Kidneys also regulate blood pressure, stimulate red blood cell production, and help maintain strong bones. When kidney health is compromised, these critical functions can be jeopardized, leading to a range of health challenges.

The Post-Transplant Recovery Journey

For those who have undergone the transformative journey of a kidney transplant, the path to recovery is a remarkable one. The surgery itself marks a significant milestone, but it's essential to understand that recovery is an ongoing process.

Following the transplant, the body requires time to adapt to the new kidney and integrate it fully. You may experience both physical and emotional changes during this phase, and it's perfectly normal to have questions and concerns.

Proper post-transplant care, including adherence to medications and lifestyle adjustments, is pivotal to ensure the long-term success of the transplant.

Harnessing the Power of Diet for Kidney Health

Diet emerges as a pivotal aspect of kidney health, even more so in the context of post-transplant recovery. A well-crafted diet can aid in maintaining optimal kidney function, preventing potential complications, and supporting overall well-being.

Kidney transplant recipients should aim for a diet that's rich in nutrients, low in sodium, and appropriately balanced. This approach helps in managing blood pressure, maintaining a healthy weight, and avoiding the strain that excessive salt intake can place on the kidneys.

Balancing Nutritional Intake

It's important to remember that the kidney's newfound lease on life after a transplant warrants attention to nutrient intake. Proteins, for instance, play a significant role in tissue repair and overall health, but excessive consumption can burden the kidneys.

Selecting high-quality protein sources, such as lean meats, poultry, fish, eggs, and legumes, can strike a healthy balance. Additionally, steering clear of foods that are high in potassium and phosphorus is crucial, as these minerals can accumulate in the blood and lead to complications.

Chapter 2: Principles of a Kidney-Friendly Diet

In this chapter, we delve into the fundamental principles of a kidney-friendly diet, a cornerstone for kidney transplant patients on their journey to wellness.

A kidney transplant is a significant milestone, and adopting the right dietary choices can greatly enhance the success of the procedure and the overall well-being of the individual.

Controlling Sodium, Potassium, and Phosphorus Intake

One of the core principles of a kidney-friendly diet is the vigilant management of sodium, potassium, and phosphorus intake.

These minerals, while essential for bodily functions, require careful regulation for those with new kidneys. Excessive consumption can lead to complications and strain on the transplanted kidney.

Sodium: Keeping an eye on sodium intake is vital as it can contribute to high blood pressure, a risk factor for kidney problems. Opt for fresh foods over processed ones, as they tend to be lower in sodium. Flavoring meals with herbs and spices, rather than salt, can add zest without compromising health.

Potassium: Proper management of potassium levels is crucial for maintaining a stable heart rhythm and preventing muscle weakness. Foods rich in potassium, like bananas and oranges, should be consumed in moderation. Instead, focus on kidney-friendly fruits and vegetables, such as apples and cauliflower.

Phosphorus: Controlling phosphorus is essential to prevent weakened bones and calcium buildup in blood vessels. Many processed foods are high in phosphorus additives, so opting for whole, unprocessed foods is key. Limiting dairy and choosing lean protein sources can also help manage phosphorus levels effectively.

Managing Fluid Balance

Fluid balance is another vital aspect of a kidney-friendly diet. The kidneys play a pivotal role in regulating the body's fluid levels, and kidney transplant patients need to be mindful of maintaining this balance. Too much fluid can strain the kidneys, while too little can lead to dehydration.

High-Quality Protein Sources

Incorporating high-quality protein sources is essential for kidney transplant patients. Protein is necessary for tissue repair and overall health, but the source matters. Lean meats like chicken and turkey, as well as plant-based options like beans and lentils, are excellent choices. These proteins provide the necessary nutrients without burdening the kidneys.

Addressing the Kidney Transplant Patients

For those who have embarked on the journey of kidney transplantation, these principles form the foundation of a nourishing diet. It's important to remember that these guidelines are not meant to be restrictive, but rather empowering.

A kidney-friendly diet offers a pathway to renewed vitality, allowing patients to savor a variety of delicious, wholesome foods while prioritizing their health.

In short, understanding and embracing the principles of a kidney-friendly diet is pivotal for kidney transplant patients. By managing sodium, potassium, and phosphorus intake, maintaining fluid balance, and selecting high-quality protein sources, individuals can pave the way for a successful and fulfilling life post-transplant.

This chapter sets the stage for the recipes that follow, each crafted with care to align with these principles and contribute to the holistic wellness of kidney transplant patients.

Remember, a kidney-friendly diet is not merely a regimen; it's a recipe for thriving with vitality and embracing the gift of renewed health.

Chapter 3: Breakfasts to Kickstart Your Day

1. Scrambled Egg and Spinach Breakfast Bowl

Prep Time: 5 minutes

Cook Time: 5 minutes

Serving Size: 1

Ingredients:

- 2 eggs

- 1 cup fresh spinach, chopped

- 1/4 teaspoon black pepper

- 1 teaspoon olive oil

Preparation:

1. In a bowl, whisk the eggs and black pepper together.

2. Heat olive oil in a non-stick pan over medium heat.

3. Add chopped spinach and sauté for 1-2 minutes until wilted.

4. Pour the whisked eggs into the pan and scramble until cooked through.

5. Serve warm.

Benefit for Kidney Transplant: This protein-rich breakfast provides essential amino acids for tissue repair after surgery. Spinach adds a dose of iron and antioxidants, supporting overall health and aiding in red blood cell formation.

2. Greek Yogurt Parfait

Prep Time: 5 minutes

Serving Size: 1

Ingredients:

- 1/2 cup plain Greek yogurt

- 1/4 cup mixed berries (blueberries, strawberries)

- 2 tablespoons chopped walnuts

- 1 teaspoon honey (optional)

1. In a glass or bowl, layer Greek yogurt, mixed berries, and chopped walnuts.

2. Drizzle honey on top if desired.

Benefit for Kidney Transplant: Greek yogurt provides a creamy protein source with lower potassium content compared to regular yogurt. Berries offer vitamins and antioxidants, while walnuts add healthy fats and omega-3s.

3. Oatmeal with Almond Butter and Banana

Prep Time: 5 minutes

Cook Time: 5 minutes

Serving Size: 1

Ingredients:

- 1/2 cup old-fashioned oats

- 1 cup water

- 1 tablespoon almond butter

- 1 small banana, sliced

Preparation:

1. In a pot, bring water to a boil and add oats.

2. Cook oats until desired consistency is reached, stirring occasionally.

3. Transfer oatmeal to a bowl, top with almond butter and banana slices.

Benefit for Kidney Transplant: Oats are a good source of fiber and provide sustained energy. Almond butter adds healthy fats, while bananas offer potassium in controlled amounts.

4. Avocado Toast with Poached Egg

Prep Time: 10 minutes

Cook Time: 5 minutes

Serving Size: 1

Ingredients:

- 1 slice whole grain bread, toasted

- 1/2 avocado, mashed

- 1 egg

- 1 teaspoon vinegar (for poaching)

Preparation:

1. Poach the egg: Bring water to a simmer in a pot, add vinegar. Crack the egg into a bowl, then gently slide it into the simmering water. Cook for about 3 minutes.

2. Spread mashed avocado on toasted bread.

3. Place the poached egg on top.

Benefit for Kidney Transplant: This breakfast combines healthy fats from avocado and protein from the egg, aiding in healing and muscle recovery while keeping potassium in check.

5. Quinoa Breakfast Bowl

Prep Time: 5 minutes

Cook Time: 15 minutes

Serving Size: 1

Ingredients:

- 1/2 cup cooked quinoa

- 1/4 cup low-fat cottage cheese

- 1/4 cup diced mango

- 1 tablespoon chopped almonds

Preparation:

1. In a bowl, mix cooked quinoa and cottage cheese.

2. Top with diced mango and chopped almonds.

Benefit for Kidney Transplant: Quinoa is a complete protein with all essential amino acids. Cottage cheese adds additional protein while being lower in sodium than some other dairy options.

6. Smoothie Bowl

Prep Time: 5 minutes

Serving Size: 1

Ingredients:

- 1 frozen banana

- 1/2 cup frozen mixed berries

- 1/2 cup spinach

- 1/2 cup unsweetened almond milk

- 1 tablespoon chia seeds

Preparation:

1. Blend frozen banana, mixed berries, spinach, and almond milk until smooth.

2. Pour the smoothie into a bowl and top with chia seeds.

Benefit for Kidney Transplant: This refreshing bowl is rich in vitamins, minerals, and antioxidants, supporting overall health and kidney function.

7. Low-Sodium Breakfast Burrito

Prep Time: 10 minutes

Cook Time: 5 minutes

Serving Size: 1

Ingredients:

- 1 whole wheat tortilla

- 1 scrambled egg

- 1/4 cup black beans (low-sodium, drained)

- 2 tablespoons salsa

- 2 tablespoons diced avocado

Preparation:

1. Warm the tortilla in a dry pan or microwave.

2. Fill with scrambled egg, black beans, salsa, and diced avocado.

3. Roll up the tortilla and enjoy.

Benefit for Kidney Transplant: This burrito offers a balance of protein and fiber with controlled sodium content. Black beans provide plant-based protein and fiber for digestive health.

8. Cottage Cheese Pancakes

Prep Time: 10 minutes

Cook Time: 10 minutes

Serving Size: 2-3 pancakes

Ingredients:

- 1/2 cup low-fat cottage cheese

- 2 eggs

- 1/4 cup whole wheat flour

- 1/2 teaspoon baking powder

- 1/2 teaspoon vanilla extract

Preparation:

1. In a blender, blend cottage cheese and eggs until smooth.

2. Add whole wheat flour, baking powder, and vanilla extract. Blend again.

3. Heat a non-stick skillet over medium heat. Pour batter to make pancakes.

4. Cook until bubbles form on the surface, then flip and cook the other side.

Benefit for Kidney Transplant: These pancakes offer a protein boost with reduced sodium content. They are a tasty alternative to traditional pancakes.

9. Rice Cake with Tuna and Cucumber

Prep Time: 5 minutes

Serving Size: 1

Ingredients:

- 1 rice cake

- 1/4 cup canned tuna (in water), drained

- 1/4 cup cucumber, thinly sliced

- 1 teaspoon lemon juice

- Fresh dill (optional)

Preparation:

1. Mix canned tuna with cucumber slices and lemon juice.

2. Spread the mixture on top of the rice cake.

3. Garnish with fresh dill if desired.

Benefit for Kidney Transplant: This light and protein-rich option is low in sodium and offers a good source of omega-3 fatty acids from tuna.

10. Apple and Peanut Butter Toast

Prep Time: 5 minutes

Serving Size: 1

Ingredients:

- 1 slice whole grain bread, toasted

- 1 tablespoon natural peanut butter

- 1/2 apple, thinly sliced

Preparation:

1. Spread peanut butter on the toasted bread.

2. Arrange apple slices on top.

Benefit for Kidney Transplant: This simple and satisfying option provides a combination of fiber, healthy fats, and vitamins from both peanut butter and apples.

11. Grilled Salmon Salad

Prep Time: 15 minutes

Cook Time: 10 minutes

Serving Size: 2

Ingredients:

- 2 salmon fillets

- Mixed salad greens

- Cherry tomatoes, halved

- Cucumber, sliced

- Red onion, thinly sliced

- Olive oil

- Lemon juice

- Fresh dill, chopped

Preparation:

1. Preheat the grill and season the salmon fillets with olive oil, salt, and pepper.

2. Grill the salmon for about 4-5 minutes on each side until cooked through.

3. In a bowl, combine the salad greens, cherry tomatoes, cucumber, and red onion.

4. Whisk together olive oil, lemon juice, and chopped dill to make the dressing.

5. Top the salad with grilled salmon and drizzle with the dressing.

Benefits for Kidney Transplant: Salmon is rich in omega-3 fatty acids that support heart and kidney health. The salad provides essential nutrients and antioxidants for post-transplant recovery.

12. Lentil and Vegetable Soup

Prep Time: 10 minutes

Cook Time: 30 minutes

Serving Size: 4

Ingredients:

- 1 cup green lentils, rinsed

- Carrots, diced

- Celery, diced

- Onion, chopped

- Garlic, minced

- Low-sodium vegetable broth

- Spinach leaves

- Turmeric

- Cumin

- Black pepper

Preparation:

1. In a pot, sauté onion, garlic, carrots, and celery until softened.

2. Add lentils, turmeric, cumin, and black pepper, and sauté for a minute.

3. Add the vegetable broth and heat it until it starts boiling. Lower the temperature and allow it to gently simmer for around 25 minutes.

4. Include some spinach leaves and cook them until they become soft and droopy.

5. Serve the soup warm.

Benefits for Kidney Transplant: Lentils are an excellent source of plant-based protein and fiber, promoting kidney function and aiding digestion. The soup is low in sodium and rich in nutrients.

13. Quinoa Stuffed Bell Peppers

Prep Time: 15 minutes

Cook Time: 25 minutes

Serving Size: 3

Ingredients:

- Bell peppers, halved and seeds removed

- Cooked quinoa

- Black beans, drained and rinsed

- Corn kernels

- Diced tomatoes

- Cumin

- Paprika

- Shredded low-fat cheese (optional)

Preparation:

1. Preheat the oven to 375°F (190°C).

2. In a bowl, mix cooked quinoa, black beans, corn, diced tomatoes, cumin, and paprika.

3. Stuff the bell pepper halves with the quinoa mixture.

4. Place the stuffed peppers in a baking dish and bake for 20-25 minutes.

5. Top with shredded cheese if desired and bake for an additional 5 minutes.

Benefits for Kidney Transplant: Quinoa is a protein-rich grain that aids in muscle repair and promotes kidney health. The meal contains a small amount of salt and is rich in dietary fiber.

14. Turkey and Vegetable Stir-Fry

Prep Time: 20 minutes

Cook Time: 15 minutes

Serving Size: 2

Ingredients:

- Lean ground turkey

- Broccoli florets

- Bell peppers, sliced

- Snap peas

- Low-sodium soy sauce

- Ginger, minced

- Garlic, minced

- Brown rice, cooked

Preparation:

1. In a pan, cook the ground turkey until browned. Remove and set aside.

2. In the same pan, stir-fry ginger and garlic until fragrant.

3. Add broccoli, bell peppers, and snap peas. Stir-fry until vegetables are tender.

4. Return the cooked turkey to the pan and add low-sodium soy sauce.

5. Serve over cooked brown rice.

Benefits for Kidney Transplant: **Lean** turkey provides high-quality protein without excess fat. The stir-fry is rich in vitamins and minerals that support kidney function.

15. Chickpea and Spinach Salad

Prep Time: 10 minutes

Serving Size: 2

Ingredients:

- Canned chickpeas, drained and rinsed

- Baby spinach leaves

- Red bell pepper, diced

- Red onion, thinly sliced

- Feta cheese, crumbled

- Balsamic vinaigrette dressing

Preparation:

1. In a bowl, combine chickpeas, baby spinach, red bell pepper, and red onion.

2. Toss with balsamic vinaigrette dressing.

3. Top with crumbled feta cheese before serving.

Benefits for Kidney Transplant: Chickpeas provide plant-based protein and fiber that support kidney health. The salad is low in sodium and offers a burst of flavors.

16. Baked Herb Chicken

Prep Time: 15 minutes

Cook Time: 25 minutes

Serving Size: 2

Ingredients:

- Chicken breasts, boneless and skinless

- Fresh herbs (can be rosemary, thyme, and oregano)

- Lemon zest

- Olive oil

- Garlic, minced

- Salt and pepper

Preparation:

1. Preheat the oven to 400°F (200°C).

2. In a bowl, mix minced garlic, chopped herbs, lemon zest, olive oil, salt, and pepper.

3. Rub the herb mixture over the chicken breasts.

4. Put the chicken on a baking sheet and cook in the oven for about 20 to 25 minutes.

5. Slice and serve.

Benefits for Kidney Transplant: Lean baked chicken offers protein for muscle repair. The use of herbs adds flavor without relying on excessive salt.

17. Veggie Omelette

Prep Time: 10 minutes

Cook Time: 10 minutes

Serving Size: 1

Ingredients:

- Eggs

- Spinach leaves

- Tomato, diced

- Red onion, chopped

- Bell pepper, diced

- Low-fat cheese (optional)

- Olive oil

Preparation:

1. In a bowl, whisk eggs until well beaten.

2. Heat olive oil in a pan and sauté spinach, tomato, red onion, and bell pepper.

3. Pour the beaten eggs into the pan.

4. Cook until the edges set, then add cheese if desired.

5. Fold the omelette in half and cook until the center is cooked through.

Benefits for Kidney Transplant: Eggs provide high-quality protein. The omelette is rich in vitamins and minerals from the vegetables.

18. Spinach and Mushroom Whole Wheat Wrap

Prep Time: 10 minutes

Cook Time: 5 minutes

Serving Size: 2

Ingredients:

- Whole wheat wraps

- Fresh spinach leaves

- Mushrooms, sliced

- Red onion, thinly sliced

- Hummus

- Balsamic vinegar

- Black pepper

Preparation:

1. In a pan, sauté mushrooms and red onion until tender.

2. Warm the whole wheat wraps.

3. Spread hummus on each wrap.

4. Layer with fresh spinach leaves and sautéed mushrooms and onion.

5. Drizzle with balsamic vinegar and season with black pepper.

6. Roll up the wraps and enjoy.

Benefits for Kidney Transplant: Spinach is rich in vitamins and iron, promoting kidney health. The wrap is a balanced option with whole grains and vegetables.

19. Tuna and White Bean Salad

Prep Time: 15 minutes

Serving Size: 2

Ingredients:

- Canned tuna, drained

- White beans, drained and rinsed

- Red onion, chopped

- Cherry tomatoes, halved

- Cucumber, diced

- Lemon juice

- Olive oil

- Fresh parsley, chopped

Preparation:

1. In a bowl, combine tuna, white beans, red onion, cherry tomatoes, and cucumber.

2. Whisk together lemon juice and olive oil for the dressing.

3. Toss the salad with the dressing and top with chopped parsley.

Benefits for Kidney Transplant: Tuna provides lean protein and omega-3 fatty acids. White beans add fiber for digestive health.

20. Roasted Vegetable Quinoa Bowl

Prep Time: 15 minutes

Cook Time: 25 minutes

Serving Size: 2

Ingredients:

- Mixed vegetables (such as zucchini, bell peppers, and carrots), diced

- Olive oil

- Quinoa, cooked

- Low-sodium vegetable broth

- Lemon juice

- Fresh basil, chopped

Preparation:

1. Preheat the oven to 400°F (200°C).

2. Toss diced vegetables with olive oil and roast until tender.

3. In a saucepan, heat low-sodium vegetable broth and lemon juice.

4. Add cooked quinoa and stir until heated through.

5. Serve quinoa topped with roasted vegetables and chopped fresh basil.

Benefits for Kidney Transplant: Roasted vegetables offer vitamins and antioxidants. Quinoa provides protein and fiber, promoting kidney function.

Chapter 5: Nourishing Dinners for Recovery and Wellness

21. Grilled Citrus Salmon

Prep Time: 15 minutes

Cook Time: 15 minutes

Serving Size: 2

Ingredients:

- 2 salmon fillets

- 1 lemon's zest and juice

- Zest and juice of 1 orange

- 1 tablespoon olive oil

- Salt and pepper to taste

Preparation:

1. Mix lemon and orange zest and juice with olive oil, salt, and pepper.

2. Marinate salmon in the mixture for 10 minutes.

3. Grill salmon for about 7-8 minutes on each side.

Benefit for Kidney Transplant: This recipe provides lean protein, heart-healthy fats, and a dose of vitamins from citrus fruits, supporting kidney function and overall recovery.

22. Quinoa-Stuffed Bell Peppers

Prep Time: 20 minutes

Cook Time: 30 minutes

Serving Size: 4

Ingredients:

- 4 bell peppers

- 1 cup cooked quinoa

- 1 cup cooked black beans

- 1 cup diced tomatoes

- 1 teaspoon cumin

- 1 teaspoon paprika

Preparation:

1. Preheat oven to 375°F (190°C).

2. Cut off the tops from the bell peppers and take out the seeds.

3. Mix cooked quinoa, black beans, diced tomatoes, cumin, and paprika.

4. Stuff peppers with quinoa mixture and bake for 25-30 minutes.

Benefit for Kidney Transplant: Quinoa offers complete protein and essential nutrients, while bell peppers provide vitamins and antioxidants, aiding in recovery and immune support.

23. Lemon Herb Chicken with Roasted Vegetables

Prep Time: 15 minutes

Cook Time: 25 minutes

Serving Size: 2

Ingredients:

- 2 boneless, skinless chicken breasts

- 1 lemon's zest and juice

- 2 cloves garlic, minced

- Mixed vegetables (can be zucchini, bell peppers, and carrots)

Preparation:

1. Marinate chicken in lemon zest, juice, and minced garlic for 10 minutes.

2. Roast chicken and mixed vegetables at 400°F (200°C) for 20-25 minutes.

Benefit for Kidney Transplant: Lean protein from chicken, combined with vitamin-rich vegetables, promotes tissue repair and supports kidney health.

24. Lentil Spinach Soup

Prep Time: 10 minutes

Cook Time: 25 minutes

Serving Size: 4

Ingredients:

- 1 cup green lentils

- 1 onion, chopped

- 2 carrots, diced

- 2 cups spinach

- 4 cups low-sodium vegetable broth

Preparation:

1. Sauté onion and carrots until tender.

2. Add lentils and vegetable broth, bring to a boil, then simmer for 20 minutes.

3. Add spinach and cook until wilted.

Benefit for Kidney Transplant: Lentils provide plant-based protein and fiber, aiding digestion and supporting kidney function.

25. Baked Cod with Herbed Quinoa

Prep Time: 10 minutes

Cook Time: 20 minutes

Serving Size: 2

Ingredients:

- 2 cod fillets

- 1 cup cooked quinoa

- Fresh herbs (parsley, dill, chives)

- 1 lemon, sliced

Preparation:

1. Place cod fillets on a baking sheet, top with lemon slices.

2. Bake at 375°F (190°C) for 15-20 minutes.

3. Mix cooked quinoa with chopped fresh herbs.

Benefit for Kidney Transplant: Cod is a lean source of protein, while quinoa and herbs provide essential nutrients, supporting post-transplant health.

26. Ginger-Turmeric Tofu Stir-Fry

Prep Time: 15 minutes

Cook Time: 10 minutes

Serving Size: 2

Ingredients:

- 1 block tofu, cubed

- 1 tablespoon grated ginger

- 1 teaspoon ground turmeric

- Mixed stir-fry vegetables

- Low-sodium soy sauce

Preparation:

1. Sauté tofu cubes with grated ginger and ground turmeric.

2. Put mixed vegetables and cook by stir-frying until they become soft.

3. Season with low-sodium soy sauce.

Benefit for Kidney Transplant: Turmeric's anti-inflammatory properties and tofu's protein content make this dish ideal for kidney transplant recovery.

27. Mediterranean Chickpea Salad

Prep Time: 15 minutes

Serving Size: 4

Ingredients:

- 2 cups cooked chickpeas

- Cucumber, tomato, red onion (diced)

- Kalamata olives

- Feta cheese (optional)

- Lemon juice and olive oil dressing

Preparation:

1. Mix chickpeas, diced vegetables, and olives.

2. Drizzle with Dressing made from olive oil and lemon juice.

3. Top with feta cheese if desired.

Benefit for Kidney Transplant: Chickpeas offer protein and fiber, while the Mediterranean flavors promote heart health and recovery.

28. Spinach and Mushroom Omelette

Prep Time: 10 minutes

Cook Time: 10 minutes

Serving Size: 1

Ingredients:

- 3 eggs

- Handful of spinach

- Sliced mushrooms

- Low-fat cheese (optional)

Preparation:

1. Whisk eggs and pour into a non-stick pan.

2. Add spinach, mushrooms, and cheese (if using) on one half.

3. Fold the omelette and cook until set.

Benefit for Kidney Transplant: Protein from eggs and vitamins from vegetables make this omelette a nutrient-rich option for recovery.

29. Roasted Vegetable and Quinoa Bowl

Prep Time: 15 minutes

Cook Time: 25 minutes

Serving Size: 2

Ingredients:

- Assorted vegetables (broccoli, bell peppers, carrots)

- 1 cup cooked quinoa

- Olive oil and balsamic vinegar dressing

Preparation:

1. Toss vegetables in olive oil and roast at 400°F (200°C) for 20-25 minutes.

2. Serve over cooked quinoa and drizzle with balsamic vinegar.

Benefit for Kidney Transplant: This bowl combines fiber-rich quinoa with antioxidant-packed vegetables, supporting kidney health.

30. Creamy Cauliflower Soup

Prep Time: 10 minutes

Cook Time: 25 minutes

Serving Size: 4

Ingredients:

- 1 head cauliflower, chopped

- 1 onion, chopped

- 2 cloves garlic, minced

- 4 cups low-sodium vegetable broth

- 1 cup unsweetened almond milk

Preparation:

1. Stir-fry the onion and garlic until they become see-through.

2. Add chopped cauliflower and vegetable broth, simmer for 20 minutes.

3. Blend until smooth, adding almond milk for creaminess.

Benefit for Kidney Transplant: Cauliflower provides vitamins and fiber, and almond milk adds a creamy touch to this nourishing soup.

Chapter 6: Snacks and Sides for Quick Nutrient Boosts

31. Zesty Cucumber Salad

Prep Time: 15 minutes

Serving Size: 1 cup

Ingredients:

- 1 cucumber, thinly sliced

- 1 small red onion, thinly sliced

- 2 tablespoons fresh lemon juice

- 1 tablespoon olive oil

- 1 teaspoon chopped fresh dill

- Salt and pepper to taste

Preparation:

1. In a bowl, combine sliced cucumber and red onion.

2. In a small bowl, whisk together lemon juice, olive oil, dill, salt, and pepper.

3. Pour the dressing over the cucumber and onion mixture, tossing gently to coat.

4. Chill in the fridge for a minimum of 30 minutes before serving.

Benefit for Kidney Transplant:

This refreshing salad is low in sodium and potassium, making it a great choice for kidney health. Cucumbers are hydrating and have a high water content, aiding in maintaining fluid balance post-transplant.

32. Herbed Quinoa

Prep Time: 10 minutes

Cook Time: 15 minutes

Serving Size: 1/2 cup

Ingredients:

- 1 cup quinoa, rinsed and drained

- 2 cups low-sodium vegetable broth

- 1 tablespoon chopped fresh parsley

- 1 tablespoon chopped fresh mint

- 1 tablespoon chopped fresh basil

- 1 tablespoon lemon juice

- Salt and pepper to taste

Preparation:

1. In a saucepan of medium size, heat up the vegetable broth until it starts bubbling.

2. Add quinoa, reduce heat to low, cover, and simmer for 15 minutes or until liquid is absorbed.

3. Fluff quinoa with a fork and let it cool slightly.

4. In a bowl, combine cooked quinoa, chopped herbs, lemon juice, salt, and pepper. Mix well.

Benefit for Kidney Transplant:

Quinoa is a protein-rich grain that provides essential amino acids without overloading the kidneys with excess protein. This dish is low in sodium and potassium and contributes to a balanced and nourishing post-transplant diet.

33. Baked Sweet Potato Fries

Prep Time: 10 minutes

Cook Time: 25 minutes

Serving Size: 1 cup

Ingredients:

- 2 medium sweet potatoes that have been peeled and cut into fries

- 1 tablespoon olive oil

- 1 teaspoon paprika

- 1/2 teaspoon garlic powder

- Salt to taste

Preparation:

1. Preheat the oven to 425°F (220°C) and line a baking sheet with parchment paper.

2. In a bowl, toss sweet potato fries with olive oil, paprika, garlic powder, and salt.

3. Spread the fries in a single layer on the baking sheet.

4. Bake for 20-25 minutes, turning halfway through, until fries are golden and crispy.

Benefit for Kidney Transplant:

Sweet potatoes provide essential vitamins and fiber, making them a healthy choice. Baking the fries reduces sodium content while retaining flavor. This snack provides a satisfying crunch without the excess potassium found in traditional potato snacks.

34. Hummus and Veggie Dip

Prep Time: 10 minutes

Serving Size: 2 tablespoons hummus + assorted veggies

Ingredients:

- 1 cup of canned chickpeas that have been drained and rinsed

- 2 tablespoons tahini

- 2 tablespoons lemon juice

- 1 small garlic clove, minced

- 1/4 teaspoon ground cumin

- Assorted veggies (carrot sticks, cucumber slices, bell pepper strips) for dipping

Preparation:

1. In a food processor, blend chickpeas, tahini, lemon juice, garlic, and cumin until smooth.

2. If needed, add a little water to achieve desired consistency.

3. Serve hummus with assorted veggies for dipping.

Benefit for Kidney Transplant:

Hummus is a protein-rich snack that's low in sodium and potassium. It provides a satisfying, nutrient-dense option for kidney transplant patients, promoting overall health and satiety.

35. Berry Yogurt Parfait

Prep Time: 10 minutes

Serving Size: 1 parfait

Ingredients:

- 1/2 cup low-fat Greek yogurt

- 1/4 cup of mixed berries (can be blueberries, strawberries, and raspberries)

- 2 tablespoons granola (low-sodium)

Preparation:

1. In a glass or bowl, layer yogurt, mixed berries, and granola.

2. Repeat the layers if desired.

Benefit for Kidney Transplant:

Greek yogurt is a good source of high-quality protein with lower potassium content compared to some other dairy products. Berries add antioxidants and vitamins, while low-sodium granola provides crunch and fiber.

36. Rice Paper Veggie Rolls

Prep Time: 20 minutes

Serving Size: 2 rolls

Ingredients:

- 4 rice paper sheets

- 1 cup mixed veggies (carrots, cucumber, bell peppers, lettuce)

- Fresh herbs (mint, cilantro)

- Low-sodium dipping sauce (soy sauce or tamari)

Preparation:

1. Prepare a shallow dish with warm water.

2. Dip a rice paper sheet into the water for a few seconds until softened.

3. Place the rice paper on a clean surface and layer with veggies and herbs.

4. Roll tightly, tucking in the sides, to form a spring roll.

5. Repeat with the remaining ingredients.

6. Serve with low-sodium dipping sauce.

These rolls are light and hydrating, offering a variety of vegetables while being low in sodium and potassium. The fresh herbs introduce flavor and antioxidants.

37. Cottage Cheese and Pineapple Bowl

Prep Time: 5 minutes

Serving Size: 1 bowl

Ingredients:

- 1/2 cup low-fat cottage cheese

- 1/2 cup fresh pineapple chunks

Preparation:

1. In a bowl, combine cottage cheese and pineapple.

Benefit for Kidney Transplant:

Cottage cheese is a protein source that's lower in potassium compared to some other dairy products. Pineapple adds a burst of flavor and provides vitamin C without excessive potassium.

38. Steamed Asparagus Spears

Prep Time: 5 minutes

Cook Time: 5 minutes

Serving Size: 5 spears

Ingredients:

- 1 bunch asparagus, tough ends trimmed

- 1 teaspoon olive oil

- Lemon zest (optional)

- Salt and pepper to taste

Preparation:

1. Steam asparagus spears until tender-crisp, about 4-5 minutes.

2. Drizzle with olive oil, lemon zest (if using), salt, and pepper.

Benefit for Kidney Transplant:

Asparagus is a nutrient-rich vegetable with minimal potassium content. Steaming preserves its natural goodness while avoiding excess sodium.

39. Almond Butter Apple Slices

Prep Time: 5 minutes

Serving Size: 1 apple

Ingredients:

- 1 apple, sliced

- 2 tablespoons almond butter (low-sodium)

Preparation:

1. Arrange apple slices on a plate.

2. Dip in almond butter before each bite.

Benefit for Kidney Transplant:

Almond butter provides healthy fats and protein without the sodium found in many traditional spreads. Apples contribute fiber and vitamins.

40. Roasted Chickpeas

Prep Time: 5 minutes

Cook Time: 25 minutes

Serving Size: 1/4 cup

Ingredients:

- 1 can chickpeas, drained, rinsed, and dried

- 1 tablespoon olive oil

- 1 teaspoon ground cumin

- 1/2 teaspoon paprika

- 1/4 teaspoon garlic powder

- Salt to taste

Preparation:

1. Preheat the oven to 400°F (200°C) and line a baking sheet with parchment paper.

2. Toss chickpeas with olive oil, cumin, paprika, garlic powder, and salt.

3. Spread chickpeas in a single layer on the baking sheet.

4. Roast for 20-25 minutes, shaking the pan occasionally, until chickpeas are crispy.

Benefit for Kidney Transplant:

Chickpeas are a protein-packed snack with moderate potassium content. Roasting them provides a satisfying crunch without the need for excess sodium.

Chapter 7: Hydration and Refreshing Beverages

41. Citrus Mint Infusion

Prep Time: 5 minutes

Serving Size: 1

Ingredients:

- 1 lemon, sliced

- 1 lime, sliced

- 5-6 fresh mint leaves

- Ice cubes

- Water

Preparation:

1. Fill a pitcher with ice cubes.

2. Add lemon and lime slices along with fresh mint leaves.

3. Fill the pitcher with water.

4. Allow the flavors to infuse for about 10 minutes before enjoying.

Benefit for Kidney Transplant: This hydrating blend of citrus and mint provides a burst of refreshing flavor while encouraging proper hydration, which is essential for supporting kidney function.

42. Cucumber Basil Cooler

Prep Time: 5 minutes

Serving Size: 1

Ingredients:

- ½ cucumber, sliced

- 4-5 fresh basil leaves

- Water

Preparation:

1. Place cucumber slices and fresh basil leaves in a glass.

2. Fill the glass with water.

3. Let the mixture sit for a few minutes to infuse the flavors.

4. Stir and sip for a cool and revitalizing drink.

Benefit for Kidney Transplant: Cucumber is hydrating and low in potassium, making it a kidney-friendly choice. Basil adds a refreshing twist and is rich in antioxidants.

43. Berry Blast Infusion

Prep Time: 5 minutes

Serving Size: 1

Ingredients:

- ½ cup mixed berries (blueberries, raspberries, strawberries)

- A few fresh rosemary sprigs

- Water

Preparation:

1. Place mixed berries and rosemary sprigs in a glass.

2. Add water and gently muddle the berries to release their flavors.

3. Allow the mixture to sit for a while before enjoying.

Benefit for Kidney Transplant: Berries are low in potassium and packed with antioxidants. Rosemary adds a unique twist and may have anti-inflammatory properties that can benefit kidney health.

44. Pineapple Ginger Refresher

Prep Time: 10 minutes

Serving Size: 1

Ingredients:

- ½ cup fresh pineapple chunks

- 1-inch fresh ginger, sliced

- Water

Preparation:

1. Combine pineapple chunks and ginger slices in a glass.

2. Fill the glass with water.

3. Let the mixture infuse for a bit before sipping.

Benefit for Kidney Transplant: Pineapple contains bromelain, an enzyme that may aid digestion. Ginger offers potential anti-inflammatory benefits, supporting overall kidney health.

45. Herbal Iced Tea

Prep Time: 5 minutes

Cook Time: 10 minutes (cooling time not included)

Serving Size: 1

Ingredients:

- 1 herbal tea bag (chamomile, hibiscus, or mint)

- Honey or stevia (optional)

- Ice cubes

Preparation:

1. Brew the herbal tea according to package instructions.

2. Allow the tea to cool completely.

3. Add honey or stevia if desired.

4. Serve over ice.

Benefit for Kidney Transplant: Herbal teas offer hydration with added benefits from their unique antioxidants. Chamomile and mint can have soothing properties, while hibiscus may help manage blood pressure.

46. Watermelon Basil Cooler

Prep Time: 5 minutes

Serving Size: 1

Ingredients:

- 1 cup fresh watermelon cubes

- 4-5 fresh basil leaves

- Water

Preparation:

1. Place watermelon cubes and basil leaves in a glass.

2. Fill the glass with water.

3. Gently muddle the ingredients to infuse the flavors.

4. Enjoy the delightful combination.

Benefit for Kidney Transplant: Watermelon is high in water content and low in potassium, making it a hydrating and kidney-friendly choice. Basil adds a burst of fresh aroma and flavor.

47. Lemon Ginger Zest

Prep Time: 5 minutes

Serving Size: 1

Ingredients:

- Juice of 1 lemon

- 1 tsp freshly grated ginger

- Honey (optional)

- Water

Preparation:

1. Combine lemon juice and freshly grated ginger in a glass.

2. Add honey if desired.

3. Fill the glass with water and stir well.

Benefit for Kidney Transplant: Lemon is a natural source of citrate, which may help prevent kidney stones. Ginger can offer anti-inflammatory and digestive benefits.

48. Minty Blueberry Splash

Prep Time: 5 minutes

Serving Size: 1

Ingredients:

- ½ cup fresh blueberries

- 4-5 fresh mint leaves

- Water

Preparation:

1. Place fresh blueberries and mint leaves in a glass.

2. Fill the glass with water.

3. Allow the mixture to sit for a while before enjoying.

Benefit for Kidney Transplant: Blueberries are rich in antioxidants and low in potassium, making them a smart choice for kidney health. Mint adds a refreshing kick.

49. Apple Cinnamon Refresher

Prep Time: 5 minutes

Cook Time: 10 minutes (cooling time not included)

Serving Size: 1

Ingredients:

- 1 apple, thinly sliced

- 1 cinnamon stick

- Water

Preparation:

1. Place apple slices and cinnamon stick in a glass.

2. Fill the glass with water.

3. Let the mixture infuse for a while.

Benefit for Kidney Transplant: Apples are a good source of dietary fiber and antioxidants. Cinnamon may have anti-inflammatory properties and can add warmth to the drink.

50. Peach Basil Elixir

Prep Time: 5 minutes

Serving Size: 1

Ingredients:

- 1 ripe peach, sliced

- 4-5 fresh basil leaves

- Water

Preparation:

1. Combine sliced peach and basil leaves in a glass.

2. Fill the glass with water.

3. Allow the flavors to meld before enjoying.

Benefit for Kidney Transplant: Peaches provide hydration along with vitamins and minerals. Basil adds a touch of herbal goodness and flavor.

Significance of Proper Hydration for Kidney Function

Proper hydration is essential for kidney function, especially for those who have undergone a transplant. Hydration helps maintain blood volume, supports waste elimination, and prevents kidney stones. Staying hydrated ensures that the kidneys can effectively filter waste and maintain electrolyte balance.

Incorporating Hydration into Kidney-Transplant Diets

These refreshing drink recipes align with the principles of kidney-transplant diets by focusing on low-sodium and low-potassium ingredients. They provide an enjoyable and flavorful way to stay hydrated, promoting overall kidney health.

By infusing beverages with herbs and fruits, these drinks offer not only hydration but also a burst of nutrients and antioxidants that contribute to the well-being of kidney transplant recipients.

Chapter 8: 7-Day Kidney Health and Recovery Meal Plan

Day 1:

- Breakfast (Recipe 3): Oatmeal with Almond Butter and Banana

- Lunch (Recipe 15): Chickpea and Spinach Salad

- Dinner (Recipe 21): Grilled Citrus Salmon

- Snack (Recipe 32): Herbed Quinoa

- Dessert (Recipe 35): Berry Yogurt Parfait

Day 2:

- Breakfast (Recipe 2): Greek Yogurt Parfait

- Lunch (Recipe 14): Turkey and Vegetable Stir-Fry

- Dinner (Recipe 22): Quinoa-Stuffed Bell Peppers

- Snack (Recipe 34): Hummus and Veggie Dip

- Dessert (Recipe 37): Cottage Cheese and Pineapple Bowl

Day 3:

- Breakfast (Recipe 8): Cottage Cheese Pancakes

- Lunch (Recipe 11): Grilled Salmon Salad

- Dinner (Recipe 23): Lemon Herb Chicken with Roasted Vegetables

- Snack (Recipe 38): Steamed Asparagus Spears

- Dessert (Recipe 39): Almond Butter Apple Slices

Day 4:

- Breakfast (Recipe 10): Apple and Peanut Butter Toast

- Lunch (Recipe 13): Quinoa Stuffed Bell Peppers

- Dinner (Recipe 26): Ginger-Turmeric Tofu Stir-Fry

- Snack (Recipe 31): Zesty Cucumber Salad

- Dessert (Recipe 36): Rice Paper Veggie Rolls

Day 5:

- Breakfast (Recipe 6): Smoothie Bowl

- Lunch (Recipe 19): Tuna and White Bean Salad

- Dinner (Recipe 24): Lentil Spinach Soup

- Snack (Recipe 33): Baked Sweet Potato Fries

- Dessert (Recipe 40): Roasted Chickpeas

Day 6:

- Breakfast (Recipe 5): Quinoa Breakfast Bowl

- Lunch (Recipe 12): Lentil and Vegetable Soup

- Dinner (Recipe 27): Mediterranean Chickpea Salad

- Snack (Recipe 44): Pineapple Ginger Refresher

- Dessert (Recipe 46): Watermelon Basil Cooler

Day 7:

- Breakfast (Recipe 1): Scrambled Egg and Spinach Breakfast Bowl

- Lunch (Recipe 18): Spinach and Mushroom Whole Wheat Wrap

- Dinner (Recipe 30): Creamy Cauliflower Soup

- Snack (Recipe 42): Cucumber Basil Cooler

- Dessert (Recipe 49): Apple Cinnamon Refresher

Importance of Following the Meal Plan

Following this 7-day meal plan tailored for kidney health and recovery is essential for optimal results. Each meal is thoughtfully crafted to align with the principles of kidney-transplant diets, providing a balance of nutrients that support kidney function, manage sodium and potassium intake, and promote overall wellness.

These meals are designed to provide sustained energy, essential nutrients, and a variety of flavors, ensuring that your body gets what it needs to heal and thrive.

The combination of these recipes not only offers delicious and satisfying meals but also contributes to your post-transplant journey. Proper nutrition can aid in faster recovery, reduce the risk of complications, and enhance the overall quality of life.

By adhering to this meal plan, you're giving your body the best chance to heal, adapt, and thrive, while enjoying a diverse range of flavorful and nourishing dishes.

Chapter 9: Tips for Success and Long-Term Kidney Wellness

Congratulations on taking the important step towards kidney health and recovery with 'The Kidney Transplant Diet Recipes Cookbook'. As you continue your journey beyond recovery, it's crucial to maintain a kidney-friendly lifestyle that supports your overall well-being and promotes long-term wellness.

This section offers practical tips for success, helping you navigate life with a thriving spirit and a nourished body.

1. Sustain the Good Habits: The recipes in this cookbook were carefully curated to align with kidney health principles. As you progress, don't view these recipes as a temporary solution.

Instead, incorporate them as a part of your daily routine. Choose whole, fresh foods over processed options, and make mindful choices that prioritize your kidney health.

2. Portion Control Matters: While the ingredients are kidney-friendly, portion control remains significant. Pay attention to serving sizes to ensure that you're not overloading your body with excessive nutrients. Consult with a healthcare professional to determine the right portions that suit your individual needs.

3. Stay Hydrated: Adequate hydration is vital for kidney function. The refreshing beverage recipes in the cookbook are designed to keep you hydrated and provide essential nutrients. Continue to prioritize hydration in your daily routine, as it supports waste elimination and overall kidney health.

4. Embrace Variety: Variety isn't just the spice of life; it's also a key principle for kidney wellness. Rotate through the recipes and explore new ingredients to ensure you're receiving a wide range of nutrients. Different foods bring different benefits to the table, enriching your diet and promoting overall health.

5. *Regular Medical Check-ups:* Your journey towards kidney health isn't a solitary one. Regular medical check-ups and consultations with your healthcare team are essential. These professionals can monitor your progress, adjust your dietary recommendations as needed, and address any concerns that may arise.

6. *Mindful Sodium Management:* The cookbook emphasizes low-sodium recipes, and that's a practice worth continuing. Too much sodium can strain the kidneys, so be cautious when adding salt to your meals. Opt for herbs and spices to enhance flavors, and read food labels to make informed choices.

7. *Monitor Potassium and Phosphorus Intake:* Kidneys play a role in balancing potassium and phosphorus levels. Keep an eye on these nutrients, and choose foods that fit within the recommended guidelines. The cookbook's recipes can serve as a foundation for understanding how to manage these elements in your diet.

8. Stress Management: Stress can impact kidney health. Alongside nutritious meals, incorporate stress-reduction techniques into your routine, such as meditation, deep breathing, and engaging in activities you love. A holistic approach to well-being can complement your dietary efforts.

9. Listen to Your Body: Your body is a remarkable communicator. Pay attention to how certain foods make you feel and any changes in your health. If you notice anything unusual, consult your healthcare provider promptly.

10. Embrace Sustainable Lifestyle Changes: This cookbook isn't just about recipes; it's about embracing a sustainable lifestyle. Beyond your recovery, these practices can form the foundation of a nourishing and fulfilling life. Embrace your journey towards long-term kidney wellness with enthusiasm and dedication.

Conclusion: Your Journey to Kidney Wellness

Unlocking Kidney Health: Key Takeaways from 'The Kidney Transplant Diet Recipes Cookbook'

As you close the pages of 'The Kidney Transplant Diet Recipes Cookbook', it's important to reflect on the wealth of knowledge and nourishing recipes you've encountered.

This cookbook is more than just a collection of culinary creations; it's a guide to transforming your relationship with food, embracing kidney health, and nurturing your overall well-being.

Let's recap the key takeaways that can empower you on your journey to improved kidney function and lasting wellness.

1. Nourishment for Recovery: The recipes in this cookbook are designed with precision, aligning with kidney health principles to aid your recovery and beyond. Each dish serves as a nutritional powerhouse, providing your body with the essential nutrients it needs to heal, thrive, and adapt.

2. *A Symphony of Flavors:* Embrace the symphony of flavors that these recipes offer. From the zing of citrus to the earthy notes of herbs, these ingredients come together to create dishes that are not only beneficial for your kidneys but also a delight to your taste buds.

3. *Sustained Hydration:* Proper hydration is the cornerstone of kidney health. The hydration-focused recipes and refreshing beverages in the cookbook are a reminder to keep your fluid levels balanced. By staying hydrated, you're supporting your kidneys in their vital roles within your body.

4. *Empowerment through Education:* This cookbook is also a source of education. As you've learned about sodium management, portion control, and nutrient balance, you're empowered to make informed choices that support your health journey.

5. *Culinary Creativity:* The recipes offer a canvas for your culinary creativity. Feel free to experiment, substitute ingredients, and create personalized versions of the dishes. As long as you stay within the kidney health guidelines, the possibilities are endless.

6. *Commitment to Wellness:* By embracing the recipes and principles of this cookbook, you're making a commitment to your well-being. This commitment extends beyond recovery—it's a dedication to sustained kidney health and overall wellness.

7. *A Journey of Support:* Remember, you're not on this journey alone. The cookbook is a testament to your commitment, and we're here to support you every step of the way. The guidance within these pages is a beacon of hope and a reminder that your health matters.

8. *Compassion for Yourself:* Improving kidney function and embracing wellness is a journey that requires patience and self-compassion. Embrace each step, celebrate your victories, and treat yourself with kindness throughout the process.

9. Your Unique Path: While the cookbook provides guidelines, your journey is unique. Listen to your body, collaborate with your healthcare team, and make adjustments that cater to your individual needs and preferences.

10. Future of Vibrant Health: As you embark on this journey, envision a future of vibrant health and well-being. The cookbook's recipes are a vehicle that can carry you towards this future, helping you achieve the vitality you deserve.

In closing, know that you possess the tools, knowledge, and recipes to support your kidney health and overall well-being. As you continue to incorporate the cookbook's wisdom into your daily life, remember that you're not just following recipes—you're embracing a lifestyle that celebrates your health and vitality.

The power to thrive is within you, and we're here to cheer you on every step of the way. Here's to your journey towards improved kidney function and a life filled with wellness and vitality.

Made in the USA
Las Vegas, NV
05 November 2024

11185975R00056